The Michigan Critical Care Handbook

13th Edition

1,000 indispensable facts, figures, and graphs for the adult ICU

Robert H. Bartlett, M.D.
Professor of Surgery and Director of
Surgical Critical Care Program,
University of Michigan Medical School,
Ann Arbor, Michigan

Scholarly Publishing Office, University of Michigan Library   Ann Arbor

Published in 2010 by The Scholarly Publishing Office
University of Michigan University Library

© 1996 Robert H. Bartlett

This edition is reprinted from the 1996 Little, Brown and Company
edition by arrangement with Robert H. Bartlett

This work is licensed under a Creative Commons Attribution
Non-Commercial 3.0 Unported License. License details are
available at http://creativecommons.org/licenses/by-nc/3.0/

ISBN 978-1-60785-208-7

Table of Contents

Introduction 1

Oxygen Kinetics 2

Oxygen Consumption/Delivery and Shock 4

Hemodynamics 6

Respiration 10

Oxygenation 12

Carbon Dioxide Removal 14

Metabolism and Nutrition 18

Renal Function 20

Fluids and Electrolytes 24

Acid-Base Status 25

Nervous System 26

Host Defenses/Coagulation 28

Host Defenses/Infection 30

Scoring Systems 32

Critical Care Drug Doses 37

Notice

The indications for and dosages of all drugs in this book have been recommended in the medical literature and conform to the practices of the general medical community. The medications described do not necessarily have specific approval by the Food and Drug Administration for use in the diseases and dosages for which they are recommended. The package insert for each drug should be consulted for use and dosage as approved by the FDA. Because standards for usage change, it is advisable to keep abreast of revised drug recommendations, particularly those concerning new drugs.

Introduction

This is truly a handbook. It contains no prose, only charts, tables, diagrams, and algorithms necessary for monitoring and managing critically ill patients. Basic knowledge of physiology, pathophysiology, medical management, and bioengineering is assumed.

Critical Care Physiology, also published by Little, Brown, provides a detailed explanation and rationale for the material in this handbook. These books were originally prepared in 1981 for students, residents, and staff caring for critically ill patients at the University of Michigan. The algorithms and axioms comprise the protocol for patient care in the surgical intensive care units at the University of Michigan Medical Center. This protocol will apply to 95% of critical care situations. Diagrams, algorithms, drug dosages, and axioms are presented dogmatically without specific references in this handbook. Background, discussion, and detailed references are presented in the *Critical Care Physiology* text.

This Handbook and the text *Critical Care Physiology* were originally published by Little, Brown (later Lippincott) in 1996. It is reproduced here by the University of Michigan Library's Scholarly Publishing Office. An updated edition will be published by the University in 2011.

Oxygen Kinetics

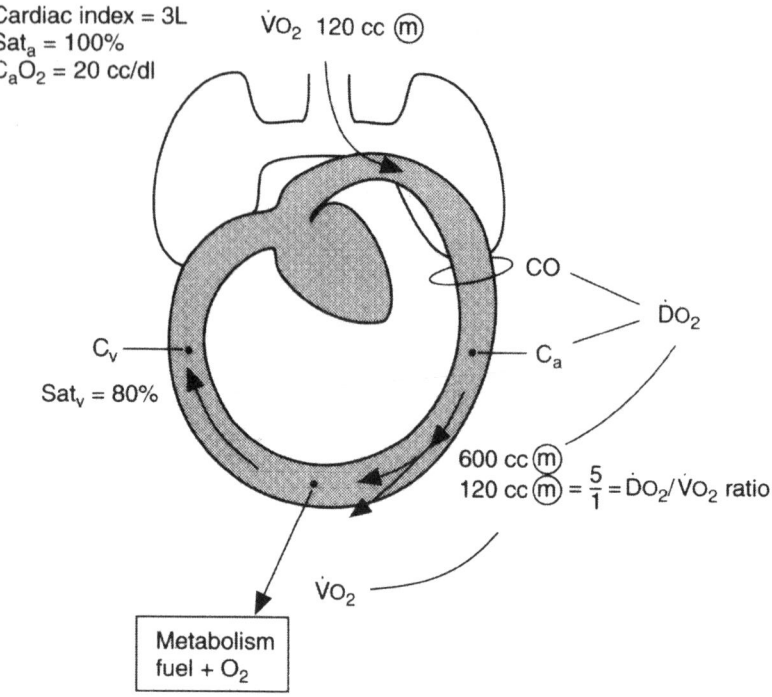

Abbreviation	Definitions	Normal value
CaO_2	Oxygen content, arterial	20 cc/dL
CvO_2	Oxygen content, venous	16 cc/dL
$AVDO_2$	Arteriovenous oxygen content difference	4 cc/dL
$\dot{D}O_2$	Oxygen delivery	600 cc/min/m²
$\dot{V}O_2$	Oxygen consumption	120 cc/min/m²
$\dot{V}CO_2$	CO_2 produced	100 cc/min/m²
REE	Resting energy expenditure	25 cal/kg/day
ⓜ	—	/min/m²

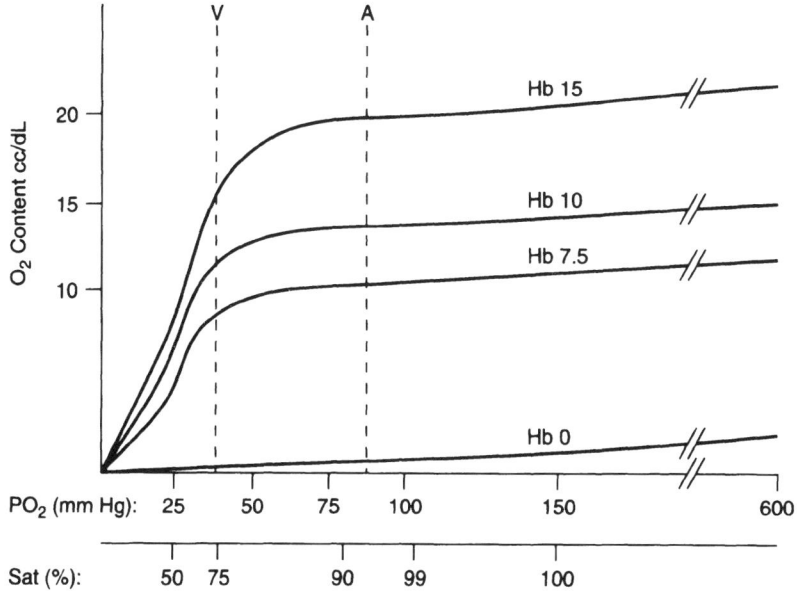

Oxygen Content = (Hb g/dL × % sat × 1.36 cc/g) + (P_{O_2} × 0.003 cc of O_2/mm Hg/dL)
Oxygen Delivery = CaO_2 × Cardiac index
Fick's axiom: O_2 consumed via lung = O_2 consumed in metabolism
CaO_2 or CvO_2 = Oxygen Content = cc of O_2/dL = O_2 bound to Hb + O_2 dissolved:
   O_2 bound to Hb = Hb g/dL × % sat × 1.36 cc of O_2/g,
   O_2 dissolved = P_{O_2} × 0.003 cc of O_2/mm Hg/dL
$AVDO_2$ = CaO_2 − CvO_2

Oxygen Consumption/Delivery and Shock

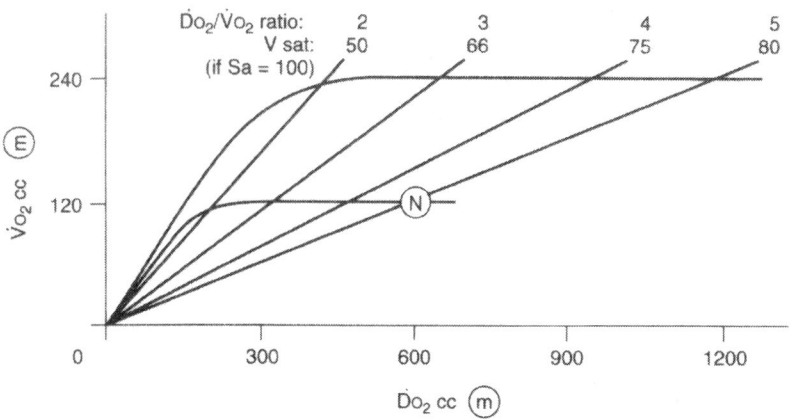

Interpreting the DO_2/VO_2 diagram

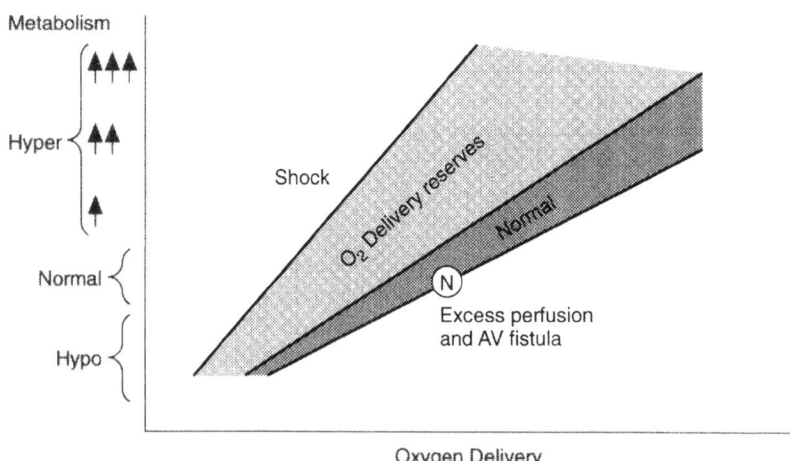

Estimating oxygen₂ delivery

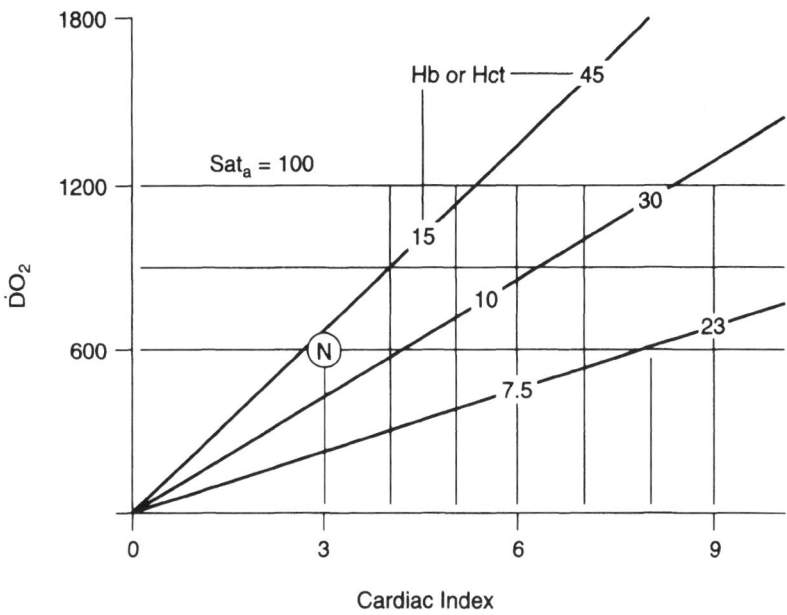

Cardiac output compensation for ① ↑ EE, ② hypoxia, ③ anemia

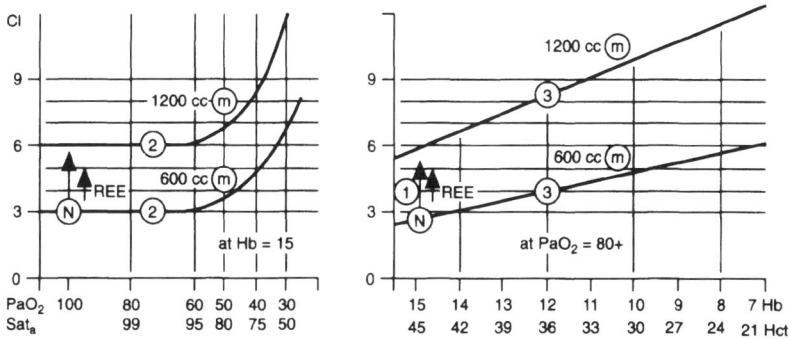

In compensation for anemia, hypoxia, or increased metabolism, cardiac output increases until DO_2 is 4–5 times VO_2. The amount of cardiac output increase required to sustain normal DO_2/VO_2 ratio is shown here for hypoxia (2), or anemia (3), during normal (N) or increased metabolism (1).

Hemodynamics

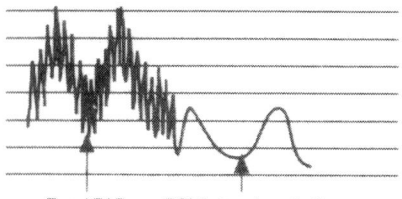

Read PAP or PCW at end-expiration

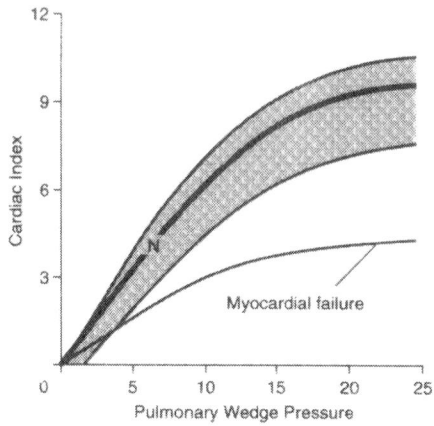

Abbreviation	Definition	Formula	Normal value
CO	Cardiac output	—	3.2 L/min/m^2
CI	Cardiac index	CO/m^2	3.2 L/min/m^2
PAP	Pulmonary artery pressure	—	25/10 mm Hg
PCW	Pulmonary capillary wedge pressure	—	5–10 mm Hg
RAP (CVP)	Right arterial pressure (central venous pressure)	—	2–5 mm Hg
BP	Systemic artery pressure	—	120/80 mm Hg
SV	Stroke volume	CO ÷ rate	
SI*	Stroke index	CI ÷ rate	45 mL/beat
SVRI*	Systemic vascular resistance index	$\frac{MAP - RAP}{CI}$	25–30 units
PVRI*	Pulmonary vascular resistance index	$\frac{MPAP - LAP}{CI}$	1–2 units
LVSWI*	Left ventricular stroke work index	SI × MAP × 0.0144	50 gm · m^{-1} · m^2
RVSWI*	Right ventricular stroke work index	SI × MPAP × 0.0144	10 gm · m^{-1} · m^2
RPP	Rate pressure product	BP × rate	12,000
Fick equation		$CO = \frac{V_{O_2}}{AVDO_2}$	

*Use CI to calculate derived variables.

Hypotension/↓ perfusion (shock) algorithm

Physical signs of shock (↓ pulse pressure, ↓ blood pressure, tachycardia, confusion, syncope)
Physical signs of venous pressure (neck veins, chest auscultation)

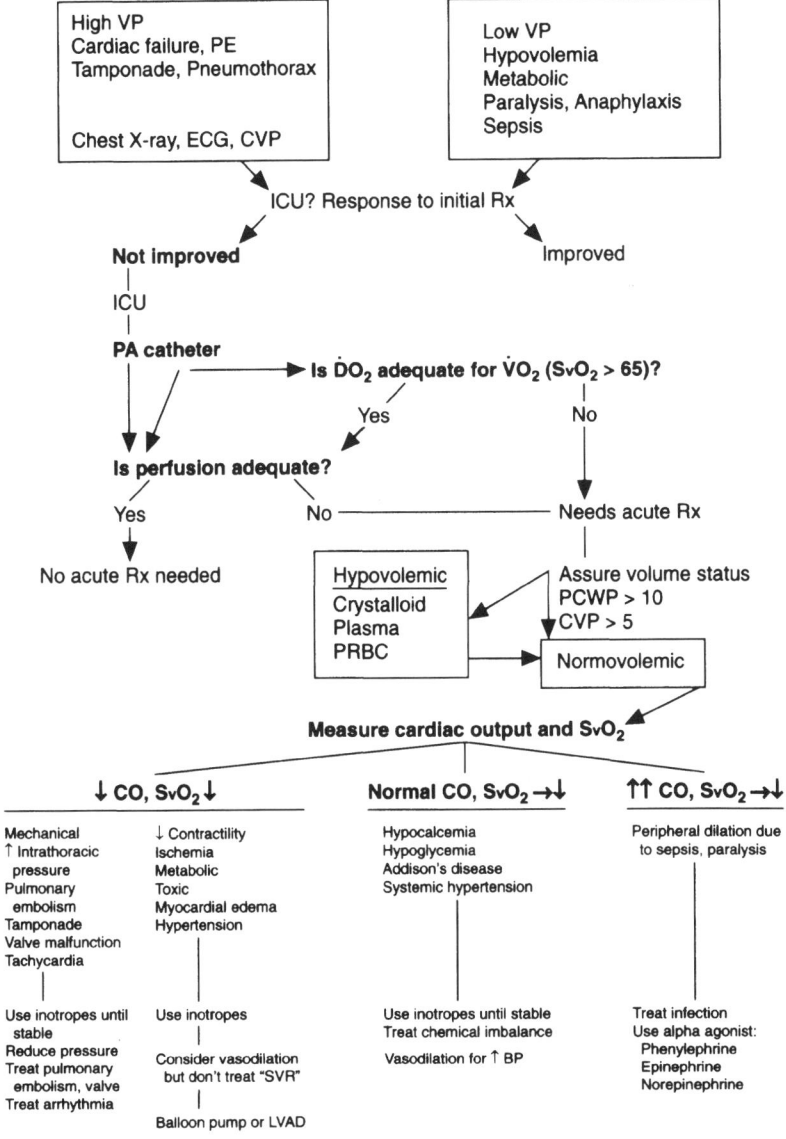

"Pressor" drugs

Drug	Contractility (Inotropic)	SA Node Rate (Chronotropic)	Vasoconstriction	Vasodilation	Renal Perfusion	Cardiac Output	Systemic Vascular Resistance	Blood Pressure	V_{O_2}, V_{CO_2}, REE
Isoproterenol	+++	+++	0	+++	↑ or ↓	↑	↓	↑↓	↑
Dobutamine	+++	0 to +	0 to +	0 to +	↑	↑	↓	0 to ↑	↑
Dopamine	+++	+	0 to +++	0	↑ or ↓	↑	↓ or ↑	0 to ↑	↑
Epinephrine	+++	+++	+++	++	↓	↑	↓	↑↓	↑
Norepinephrine	++	++	+++	0	↓	↑ or ↓	↑	↑	↑
Ephedrine	++	++	+	0 to +	↓	↑	↑ or ↓	↑	↑
Phenylephrine	0	0	+++	0	↓	↓	↑	↑	↑

REE = resting energy expenditure; SA = sinoatrial; V_{O_2} = oxygen consumption; V_{CO_2} = CO_2 production
+ = minor; ++ = moderate; +++ = major; ↑ = increased; ↓ = decreased

Inotrope algorithm

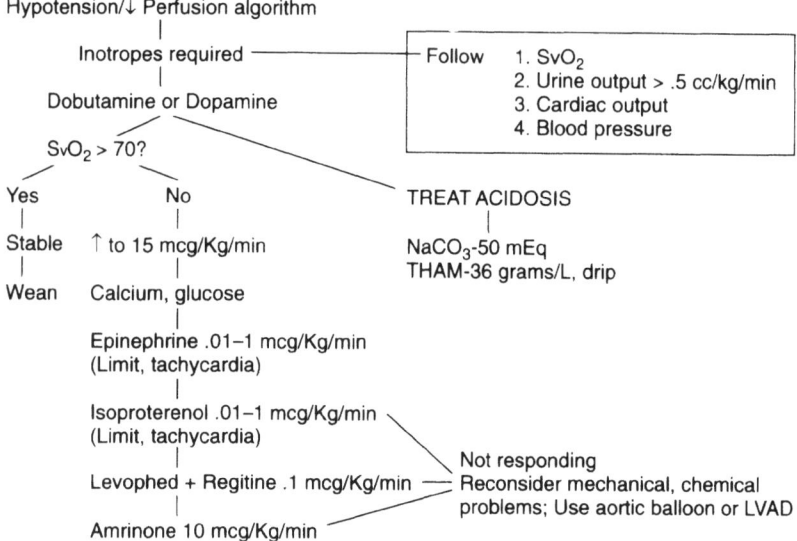

Drugs and conditions that affect the myocardial conduction system

ECG feature	Normal	↑	↓
PR interval	1.2–2	AV block	Nodal disease; WPW syndrome
QT interval	0.3–0.4	↓ Ca and ↓ Mg; lidocaine; quinidine; MI	↑ Ca, ↑ K, and ↑ Mg; digitalis
T wave	0.25 mV	↑ K, ischemia	—

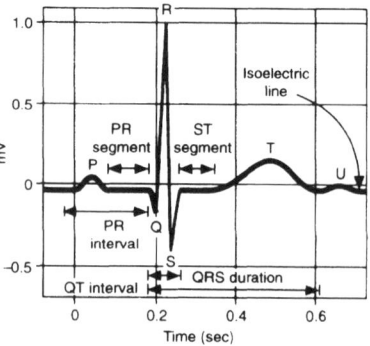

Arrhythmia Algorithms

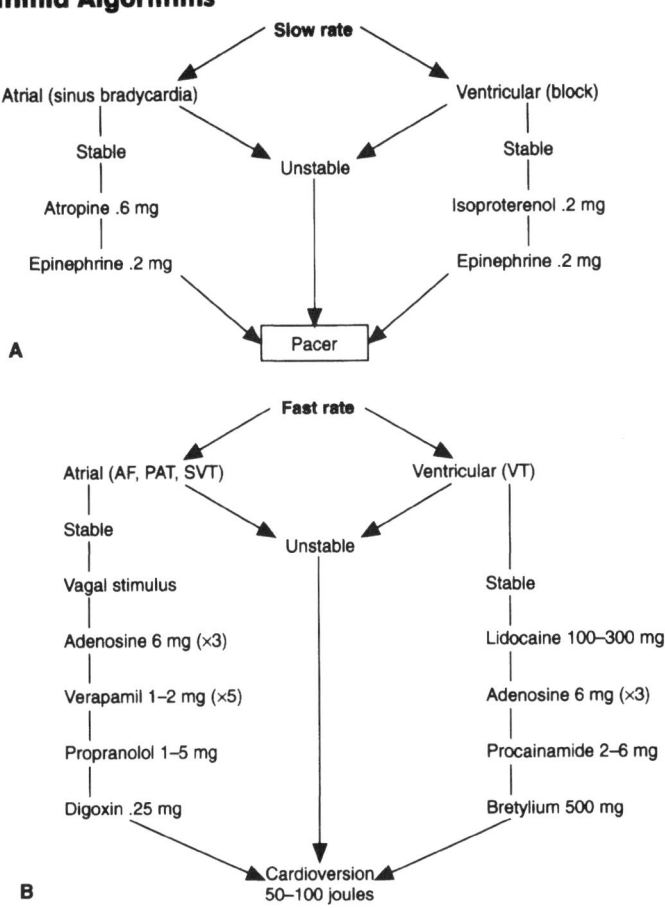

Hemodynamic Axioms

1. PCWP reflects the left ventricular filling pressure (LAP), which depends **only** on blood volume and myocardial muscle status. LAP = LVEDP if mitral valve is normal.
2. PCWP **does not** reflect extracellular fluid volume; PCWP is generally **not** related to overhydration.
3. PCWP is equal to the pulmonary artery diastolic pressure if the heart rate is < 90.
4. RAP (CVP) is always lower than PCWP, except when pulmonary vascular resistance is grossly elevated.
5. Resistance is just a calculation, not a measurement. The units are pressure per flow and mmHg per liter per minute per meter^2 (usually referred to as *Wood units*). If you multiply Wood units times 79.9, you can express resistance as dyne · sec · cm^{-5}, but why bother?
6. Use **mean** pressure and cardiac **index** to calculate derived variables (resistance, stroke index, stroke work index).
7. An elevated systemic vascular resistance index (SVRI) is almost always caused by low cardiac output, rarely by primary vasospasm. Treat the cardiac output not the "resistance."

Respiration

Pulmonary Mechanics

Abbreviation	Definition	Normal value
TLC	Total lung capacity	80 cc/kg
FRC	Functional residual capacity	40 cc/kg
IC	Inspiratory capacity	40 cc/kg
ERV	Expiratory reserve volume	30 cc/kg
RV	Residual volume	10 cc/kg
V_T	Tidal volume	5 cc/kg
V_E	Minute ventilation (exhaled)	100 cc/kg/min
V_A	Alveolar ventilation	60 cc/kg/min
V_D	Dead space	cc = weight in lbs
PIP	Peak inspiratory pressure	10 cm H_2O tidal, 40 cm H_2O max
EIP (on ventilator)*	End-inspiratory (plateau) pressure	less than PIP
EEP	End-expiratory pressure	0 cm H_2O
Compliance	V_T/EIP	2 cc/cm H_2O/kg
Effective compliance	V_T/EIP − PEEP on ventilator	1 cc/cm H_2O/kg
Resistance	Inspiratory flow/pressure	
V_D/V_T	$\dfrac{PaCO_2 - PECO_2}{PaCO_2}$	0.33

*Normal EIP value depends on ventilator settings.

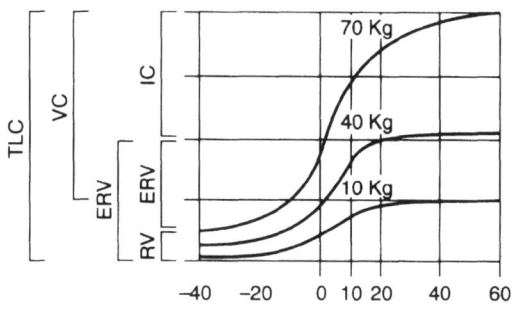

Alveolar Inflating P cm H_2O

Alveolar inflating pressure can be negative (compared to atmospheric pressure) during spontaneous breathing, or positive during mechanical ventilation. Usually, only deflation curves are shown.

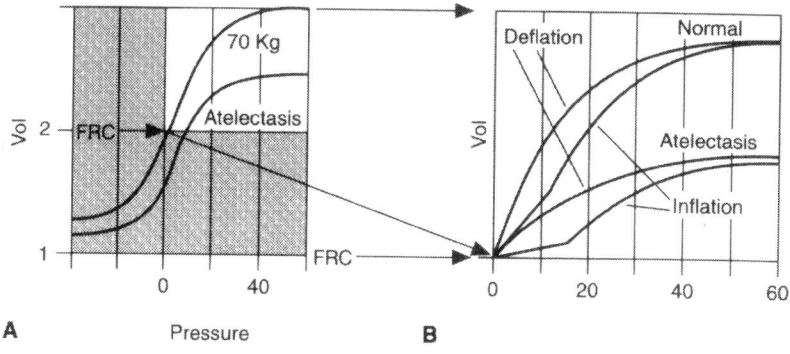

A
Compliance curves representing *deflation* from total lung capacity are shown for a normal 70-kg person and the same person with loss of alveolar volume because of atelectasis. The slope (compliance) is nearly the same for both curves, but TLC and FRC are decreased with atelectasis. Usually only the right upper quadrant of this graph is displayed, as in **B**.

B
The same deflation compliance curves as in **A**, but end expiration for each breath is plotted as zero volume, rather than true FRC. This makes the slope flatter, and the lung appears to be "stiffer." The *inflation* side of the volume-pressure curve is added to the deflation curves. In this example the inflation curve for atelectasis shows little alveolar recruitment until 16 cm H_2O is applied.

Lung volumes measured at various body positions

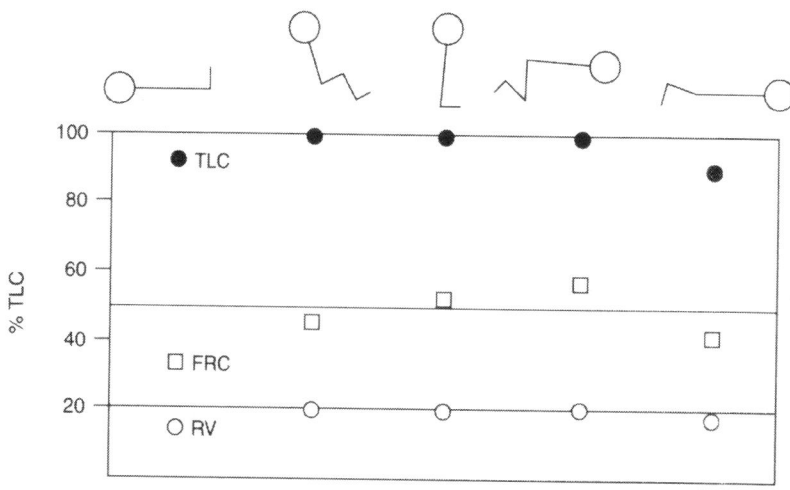

Oxygenation

Matching Blood Supply to Inflated Alveoli

Ventilation/perfusion (V/Q) Relationships

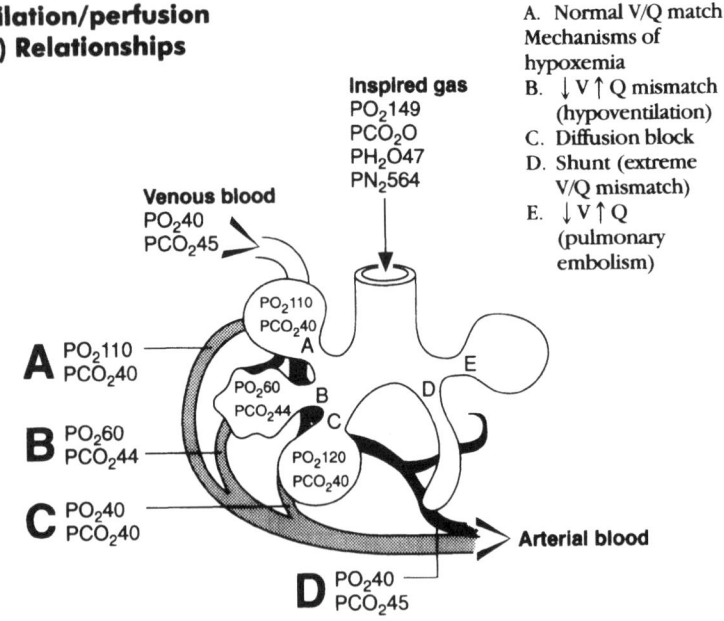

A. Normal V/Q match
Mechanisms of hypoxemia
B. ↓V ↑Q mismatch (hypoventilation)
C. Diffusion block
D. Shunt (extreme V/Q mismatch)
E. ↓V ↑Q (pulmonary embolism)

Abbreviation	Definition/Formula	Normal Value
CaO_2	Oxygen content, arterial	20 cc/dL
CvO_2	Oxygen content, venous	16 cc/dL
PAO_2	Alveolar $Po_2 = [(P_B - P_{H_2O}) \times FiO_2] - PaCO_2$	100 mm Hg (air), 673 mm Hg ($FiO_2 = 1.0$)
$AaDO_2$	Alveolar-arterial O_2 gradient: $PAO_2 - PaO_2$	10 mm Hg (air), 70 mm Hg ($FiO_2 = 1.0$)
PaO_2/FiO_2	Oxygen index (bedside shorthand)	500
CcO_2	Theoretical maximal CaO_2 at known FiO_2	22 cc/dL at FiO_2 and Hgb of 15 g/dL
% Shunt	$\dfrac{CcO_2 - CaO_2}{CcO_2 - CvO_2}$	5%

Effect of shunt on PaO₂

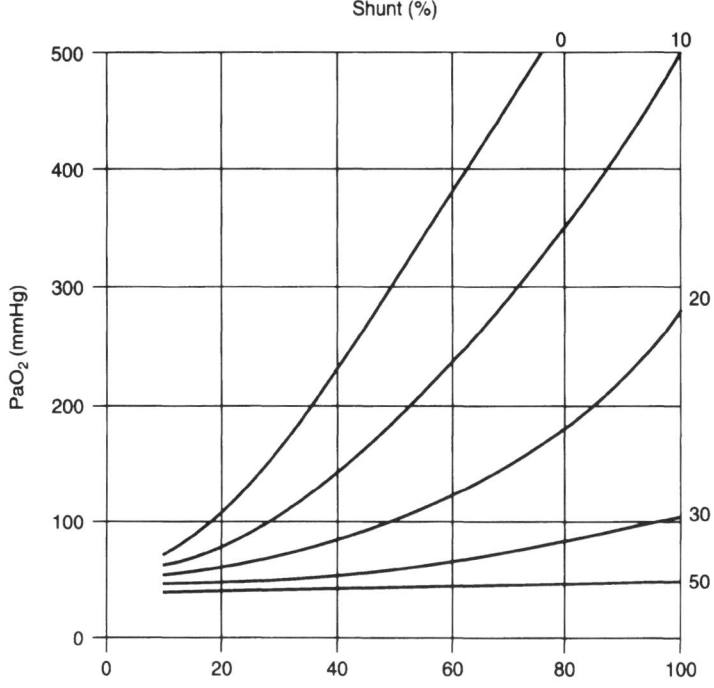

Hypoxemia as a measure of lung dysfunction

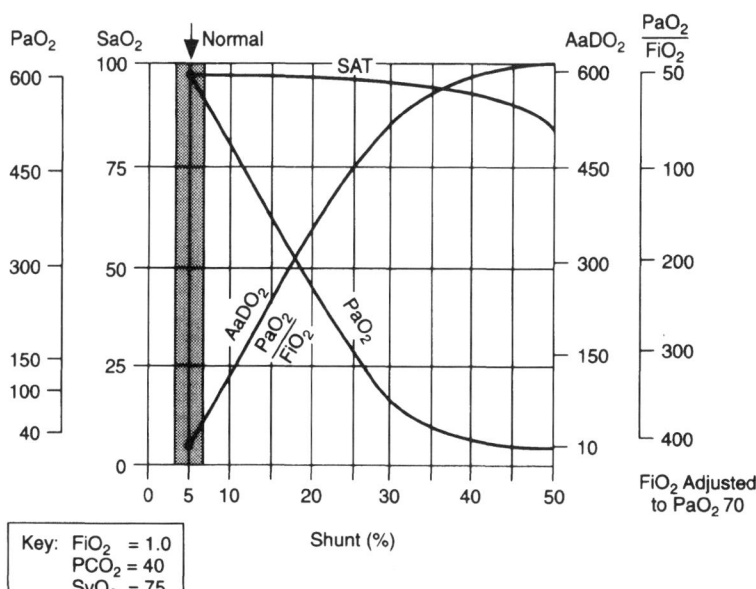

Key: FiO₂ = 1.0
PCO₂ = 40
SvO₂ = 75

Carbon Dioxide Removal

Mechanical Ventilation

Initial ventilator settings
Goal: $PaCO_2$ 40 mm Hg, SaO_2 95%
Limit: PIP 40 cm H_2O, FiO_2 0.6
TV: 10 cc/Kg or PIP: 25 cm H_2O
FiO_2: 0.5

PIP: 25 cm H_2O
PEEP: 5 cm H_2O
Flow: 60–80 LPM
Mode: Assist (backup rate 5)
Rate: 10/min if no breathing effort

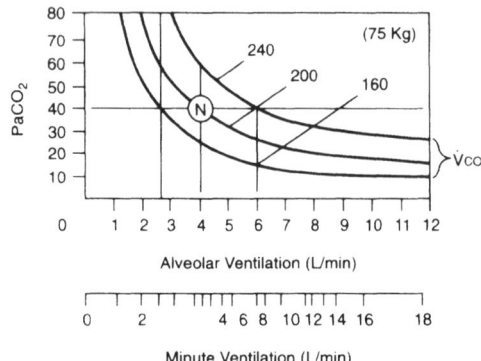

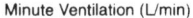

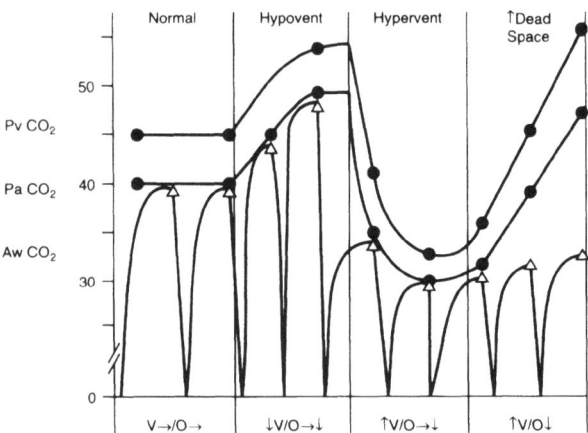

End-tidal CO_2 pressure monitoring. In this example, venous (Pv), arterial (Pa), and airway (Aw) PCO_2 are shown during various breathing patterns. The end-tidal CO_2 pressure is very close to the $PaCO_2$ as long as there is no dead space at the alveolar level. Increased alveolar level dead space (such as that caused by emphysematous bullae, honeycombing resulting from lung injury, or the exclusion of blood flow by fibrosis or low cardiac output) causes the end-tidal CO_2 pressure to be lower than the $PaCO_2$. (V/Q = ventilation-perfusion.)

Patterns of mechanical ventilation

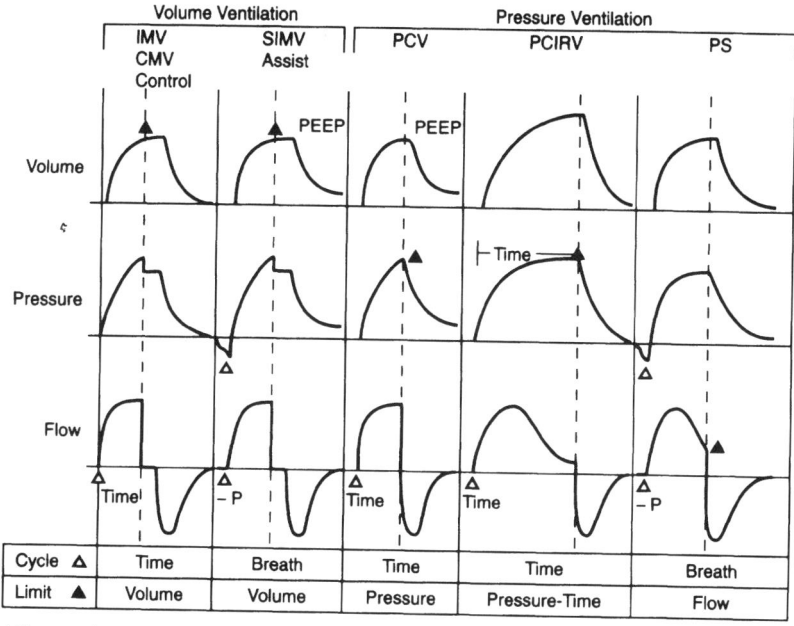

All ventilators generate gas flow which starts (cycle, control) based on a timer or triggered by patient inhalation. Gas flow stops (limit, *) when a pre-set volume or pressure or flow is reached. Volume limited ventilation should always be used with an inspiratory hold or plateau. Two examples (SIMV Assist and PCV) show the effect of PEEP. △ = start inspiratory flow; ▲ = stop inspiratory flow; IMV = intermittent mandatory ventilation; CMV = controlled, volume limited ventilation; SIMV = synchronized IMV; PEEP = positive end expiratory pressure; PCV = pressure controlled ventilation; PCIRV = pressure controlled inverse ratio ventilation; PS = pressure support.

Weaning From Mechanical Ventilation

Weaning parameters

Parameter	Result	
Inspiratory force	> 20 cm H_2O	spontaneous breathing
Tidal volume	5 cc/kg	
Vital capacity	10 cc/kg	
Minute ventilation	1 L/10 kg/min	on ventilator
SaO_2 (on FiO_2 < 0.4, PEEP < 5)	>95%	

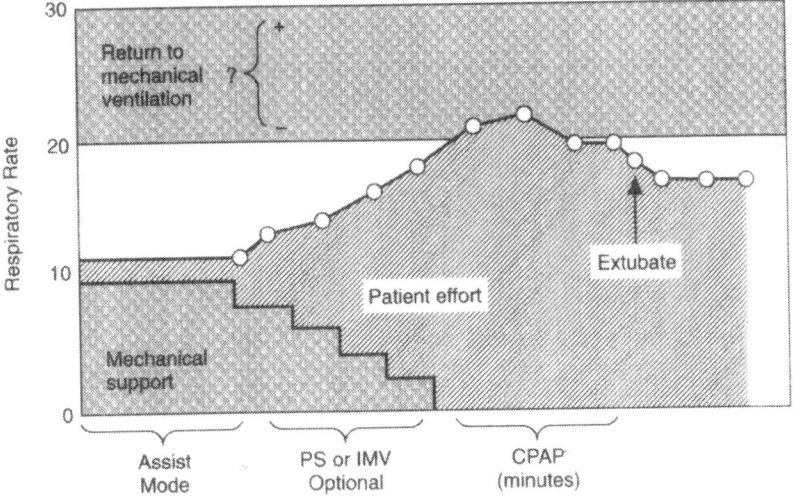

Respiratory Failure Axioms

1. Breathing and ventilation is for CO_2 removal; inflation is for oxygenation.
2. Normalize O_2 delivery, not just PaO_2.
3. Oxygenation management (FiO_2, position, suction, PEEP, and inotropes) is based on SvO_2.
4. In apnea, hypoxemia is fatal in minutes. Hypercapnia alone is "never" fatal.
5. Increasing FiO_2 decreases the alveolar nitrogen concentration and causes atelectasis.
6. Mechanical ventilation does more harm than good at high PIP and high FiO_2.
7. Never exceed EIP (plateau) of more than 40 cm H_2O. Hypercapnia is safer than EIP of more than 40 cm H_2O.
8. Ventilation management (rate, pressure, and volume) is based on the $PaCO_2$ or end-tidal CO_2 pressure.
9. Achieve and maintain dry weight.
10. Do not confuse pulmonary capillary wedge pressure with hydration status.

Respiratory failure algorithm

Acute respiratory failure (tube, ventilator, $FiO_2 > 0.5$)
(arterial catheter, oximetrix pulmonary artery catheter)

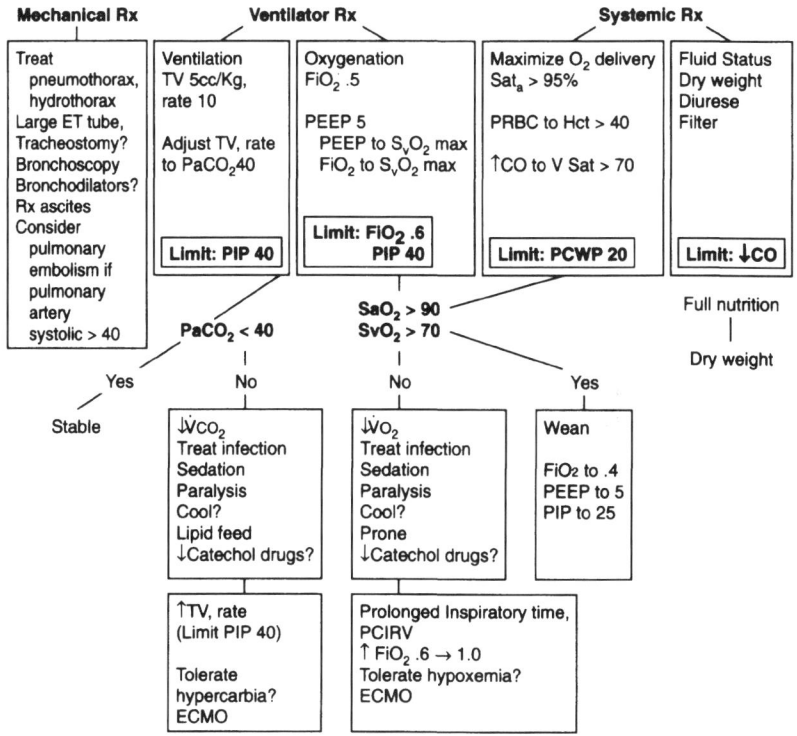

Metabolism and Nutrition

Energy
V_{O_2} = 100–130 cc ⓜ STPD
V_{CO_2} = 80–130 cc ⓜ STPD
RQ = V_{CO_2}/V_{O_2}
REE = 25 cal/kg/day; 960 cal/ⓜ/day
BEE = 20 cal/kg/day; 800 cal/ⓜ/day
Caloric balance = Calories in − REE
V_{O_2}/calorie conversion:
V_{O_2} L/min × 60 min × 24 h × 5 cal/L = cal/day
(same as V_{O_2} × 7200)

Protein
1 g of nitrogen = 6.25 g of protein
Nitrogen loss: 5–10 g/day, 85% as urea
Protein catabolic rate
 Normal: 0.5–1 g/kg/day
 Hypercatabolic = 1.5–2 g/kg/day

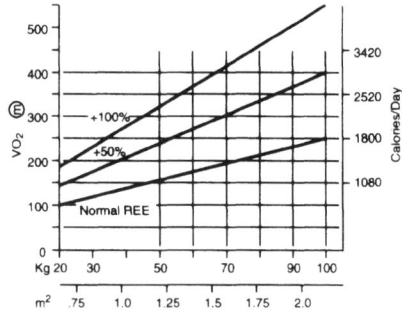

Note: Estimation of EE and PRC is often inaccurate in critically ill patients. Direct measurement is required.

Nutritional status	Depleted		Normal
Lymphocytes	< 1500	/mm³	3000
Cumulative caloric balance	− 10,000	cal	0
Cumulative protein balance	− 500	gm	0
Albumin	< 3	gm/dL	> 3
Prealbumin	< 10	mg/dL	> 20

Substrate	cal/gm	RQ	Cal/LO₂
Carbohydrate	4	1.0	5
Fat	9	0.7	4.75
Protein	4	0.8	4.8

Solution	CHO (%)	Fat (%)	Protein (%)	mOsm/L	cal/L	Na (mEq/L)	K (mEq/L)	Other
Parenteral								
10% Glucose	10	0	4.25	880	440	47	23	36 mEq acetate
25% Glucose	25	0	4.25	1825	1020	35	40	25 mEq acetate
10% Lipid	—	10	—	276	1000	0	0	—
Enteral*								
Criticare HN	22	0.3	3.8	650	1060	27	34	Tube only
Osmolyte HN	14.1	3.7	4.4	310	1060	40	40	Tube only
Isocal	12.6	4.2	3.2	300	1060	22	32	Tube only
Ensure	14.5	3.7	3.7	470	1060	37	40	Orally or tube
Jevity	15.2	3.7	4.4	310	1060	41	40	Tube only
Replete	11.3	3.3	6.2	350	1000	22	40	Orally or tube

*Commercial names are used.

Nutrition algorithm

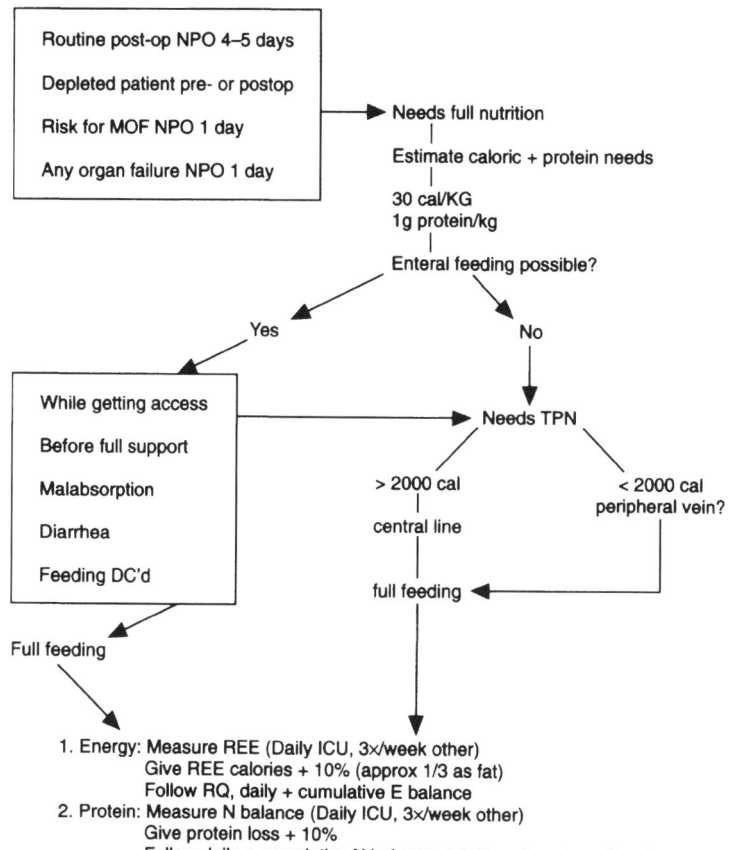

1. Energy: Measure REE (Daily ICU, 3x/week other)
   Give REE calories + 10% (approx 1/3 as fat)
   Follow RQ, daily + cumulative E balance
2. Protein: Measure N balance (Daily ICU, 3x/week other)
   Give protein loss + 10%
   Follow daily + cumulative N balance, total lymphocytes, albumin

---

Nutrition axioms

1. Estimate or measure caloric and nitrogen balance daily.
2. Use enteral nutrition whenever possible. Even small volumes prevent mucosal atrophy.
3. Treat hypoproteinemia with diuresis when appropriate, then with concentrated albumin or plasma.
4. Manage nutrition based on results of balance studies.
5. Absolute lymphocyte count and the prealbumin level are useful markers of acute-phase nutrition, but balance studies are better.
6. Tube feeding–related diarrhea can always be controlled by changing the formula, flora, or fiber.
7. Do not use antacids or H_2 blockers for stress bleeding prophylaxis. The pneumonia risk is higher than the bleeding risk.
8. When gastric pH regulation is used to treat active bleeding, measure the pH regularly and keep it over 4. Many elderly patients are achlorhydric and don't require pH control.

Renal Function

		Glomerular Filtrate		Reabsorbed %	Urine/day	
	Na	140	mEq/L	99.4	150	mEq/day
	K	5	"	Secrete	100	"
	Cl	100	"	99.2	150	"
	Urea N	15	mg/dl	50	10	gm/day
	Creat.	1	"	"O"	1.8	"
	Solute	300	mOsm/L	87	700	mOsm/day
Water	ml/min	125		99.4	.6	ml/min
	L.Hr	7.5		99.4	.04	L/Hr

→ Nephron

Abbreviation	Definition	Equation	Normal value
GFR	Glomerular filtration rate	—	2 mL/kg/min
Osm	Osmolarity/liter	—	urine = 300–1300 m Osm/L; ECF = 300 mm Osm/L
CrCl	Creatinine clearance	$\dfrac{U_{creat} \times V}{P_{creat}}$	100 mL/min
$F_E Na$	Fractional excretion of sodium	$\dfrac{U_{Na} \times P_{creat}}{P_{Na} \times U_{creat}}$	< 1%
$F_E Urea$	Fractional excretion of urea	$\dfrac{U_{urea} \times P_{creat}}{P_{urea} \times U_{creat}}$	> 50%

Drug dosage in renal failure

1. Give usual loading dose.
2. Measure or estimate creatinine clearance (C_{creat}).
3. Look up dosing line (A–H) for chosen antibiotic: e.g., gentamicin is line A.
4. Read dose fraction from graph at that C_{creat}.
5. Dose fraction times dose for patients with normal renal function per 24 hours equals maintenance dose per 24 hours.
6. Choose dosing interval you deem appropriate.
7. Additional doses may be required if patient needs hemodialysis.

Acyclovir, B
Amikacin, A
Amphotericin-B, G
Ampicillin, B
Carbenicillin, B
Cefamandole, B
Cefazolin, A
Cefotaxime, D
Cefotixin, A
Cephalexin, A
Cephalothin, A
Chloramphenicol, G
Clindamycin, G
Cloxacillin, F
Clostimethate, B
Dicloxacillin, E
Doxycycline, H
Erythromycin, D
Gentamicin, A
Ketoconazole, H
Methicillin, B
Metronidazole, G
Moxalactam, B
Nafcillin, D
Oxacillin, F
Penicillin-G, B
Piperacillin, D
Streptomycin, A
Sulfamethoxazole, E
Sulfisoxazole, F
Ticarcillin, B
Tobramycin, A
Trimethoprim, F
Vancomycin, A

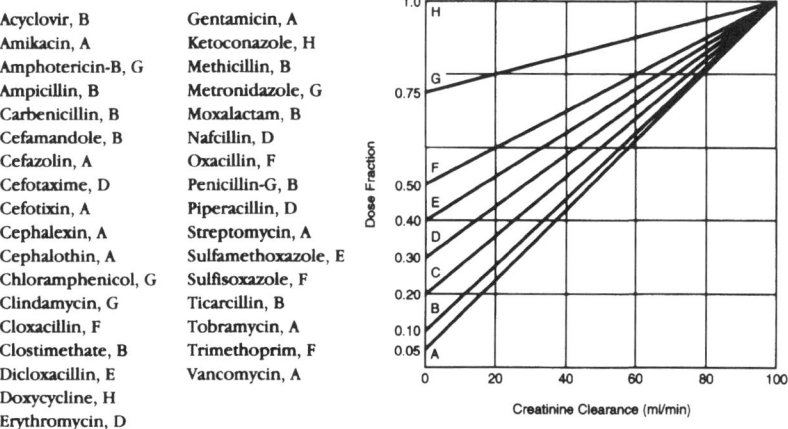

Adapted with permission from *Clin Nephrol* 1977;7:81.

Renal failure axioms

1. Clearances can be calculated using any timed urine sample; 24-hour collections are ideal but not necessary.
2. A diuretic trial is indicated if renal parenchymal disease is suspected. Use a large dose.
3. Renal failure is easy to detect but hard to admit.
4. **Full nutrition** is the systemic treatment for acute renal failure. Don't go without protein.
5. When planning renal replacement therapy, managing the extracellular fluid volume and solute toxicity are parallel but separate goals.

Acute renal failure management algorithm

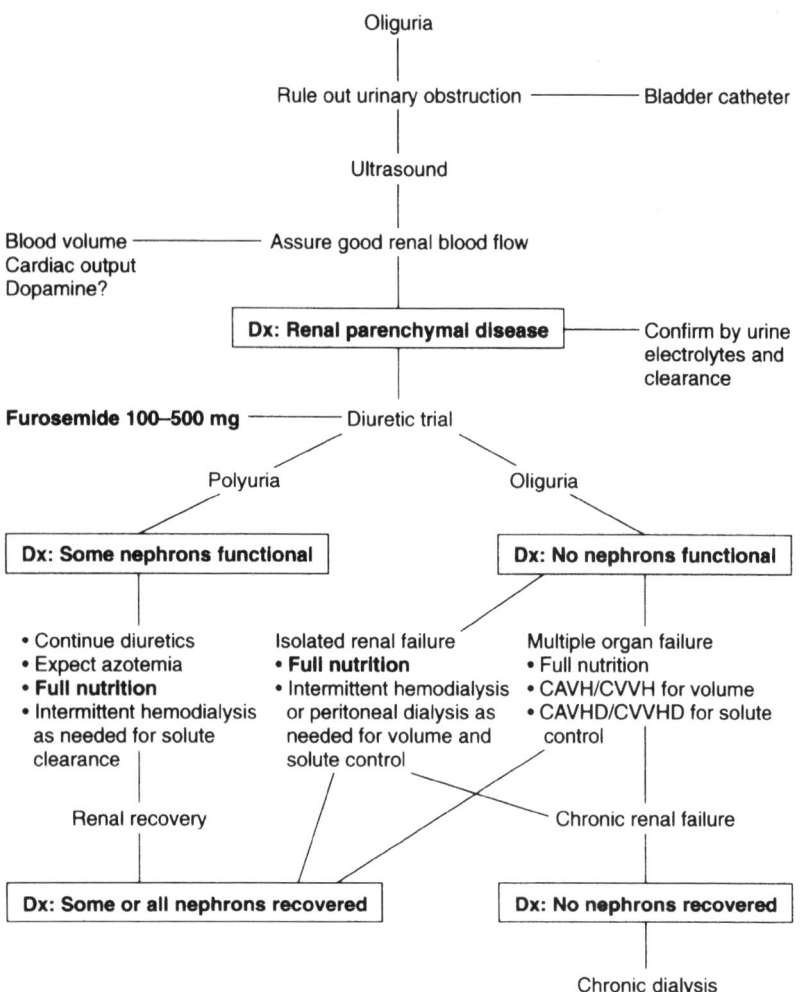

Hemofiltration

Continuous hemofiltration (CAVH, CVVH)

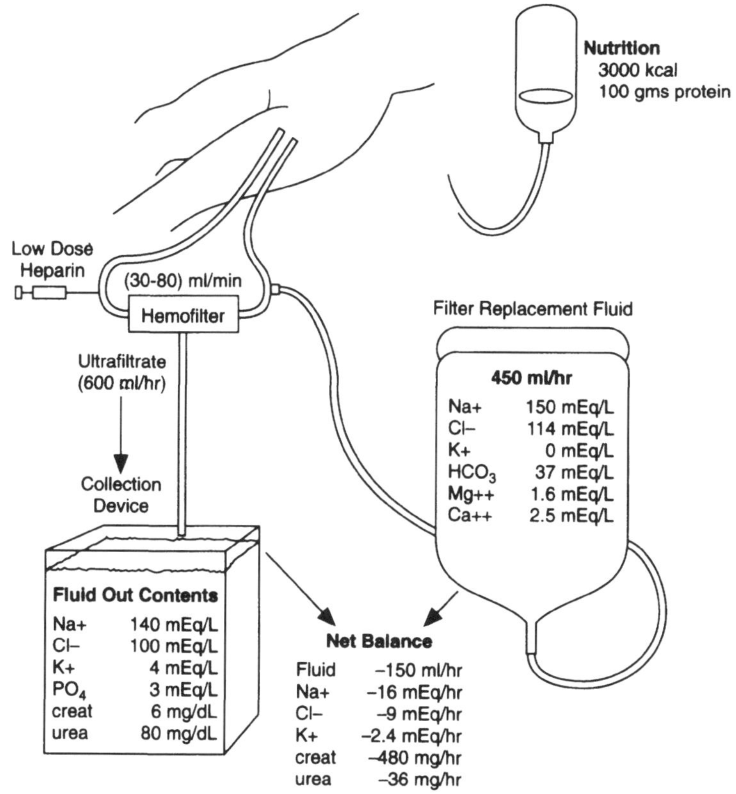

Nutrition
3000 kcal
100 gms protein

Low Dose Heparin

(30-80) ml/min
Hemofilter

Ultrafiltrate (600 ml/hr)

Collection Device

Filter Replacement Fluid

450 ml/hr
Na+	150 mEq/L
Cl–	114 mEq/L
K+	0 mEq/L
HCO$_3$	37 mEq/L
Mg++	1.6 mEq/L
Ca++	2.5 mEq/L

Fluid Out Contents
Na+	140 mEq/L
Cl–	100 mEq/L
K+	4 mEq/L
PO$_4$	3 mEq/L
creat	6 mg/dL
urea	80 mg/dL

Net Balance
Fluid	–150 ml/hr
Na+	–16 mEq/hr
Cl–	–9 mEq/hr
K+	–2.4 mEq/hr
creat	–480 mg/hr
urea	–36 mg/hr

Continuous hemodiafiltration (CVVHD)

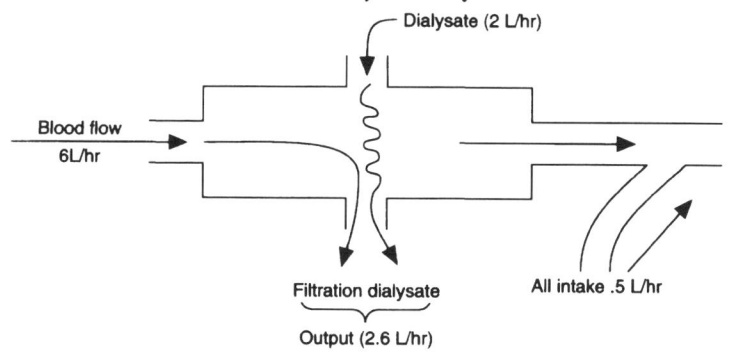

Dialysate (2 L/hr)
Blood flow 6L/hr
Filtration dialysate
Output (2.6 L/hr)
All intake .5 L/hr
Balance = –100 cc/hr, 2.4 L/day

Fluids and Electrolytes

Body composition

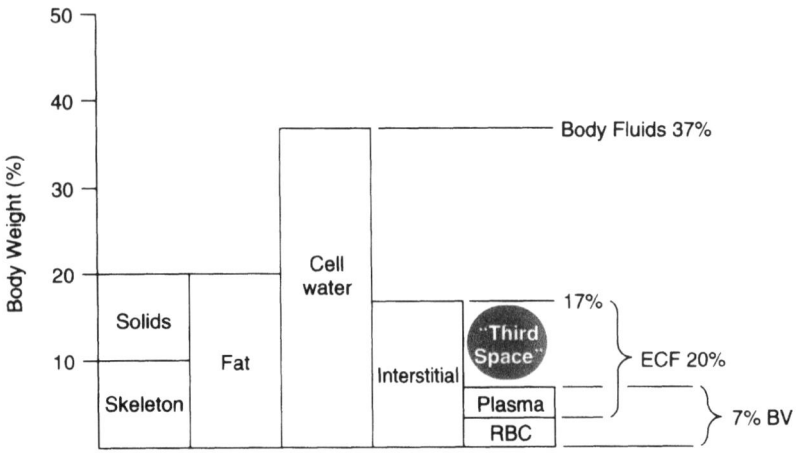

Daily requirements	H_2O	Na (mEq/L)	K (mEq/L)	Cl (mEq/L)	Calories	Protein (g/L)	Other (mEq/L)
per Kg	30	1	.5	.75	25	1g	—
50 Kg	1500	50	25	37	1250	50	—
75 Kg	2250	75	37	50	1875	75	—
100 Kg	3000	100	50	75	2500	100	—

Extracellular fluids

Gastric	20–120	15	130			H^+ 60
Bile	140	5	140			HCO_3^-, 44
Pancreatic	140	5	70			HCO_3^-, 70
Ileostomy	120	20	100			HCO_3^-, 40
Diarrhea	100	40	100			HCO_3^-, 40

IV fluids				Glucose (g/L)		Other
D5 .9 NaCl	154	0	154	50	0	600 mOsm/L
D5 ½ NS (D5 .45NaCl)	77	0	77	50	0	450 mOsm/L
Hartman (D5 LR)	130	4	109	50	—	Lactate 28, Ca 3
Standard TPN	35	40	53	250	4.25	Acetate 25, 1825 mOsm/L
Peripheral TPN	47	23	35	100	4.25	Acetate 36, 880 mOsm/L
.1 Normal HCl	••		100			H^+ 100

Acid-Base Status

Anion gap $(Na + K) - (Cl + HCO_3)$
= 12–16 > 16 = Metabolic acidosis

Buffer base deviation $27 - HCO_3$
Normal = 0
Positive = Metabolic alkalosis
(or compensated respiratory acidosis)
Negative = Metabolic acidosis
(or compensated respiratory alkalosis)

Treating buffer base deviation
Metabolic acidosis (Rx perfusion, hypoxia first):
 mEq $NaHCO_3$ required = BBD mEq/L × weight/4
Metabolic alkalosis (Rx for ventilator weaning):
 mEqHCL required = BBD mEq/L × weight/4
 (weight/4 = High estimation of ECF volume)

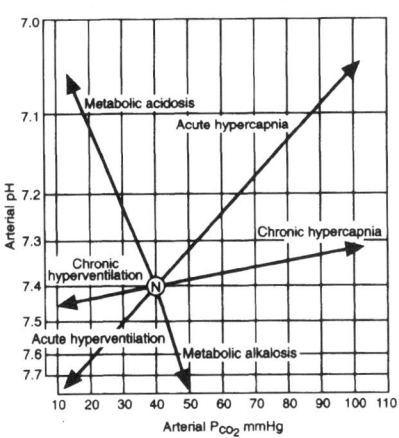

Fluid and electrolyte management algorithm (75 Kg estimated dry weight) typical example

1. Calculate requirements for 24 hours

	H₂O	Sodium (Na)	Potassium (K)	Chloride (Cl)	Calories	Protein	Example
Basic daily maintenance	2250	75	37	60	1875	75	Urine and insensible
Deficit replacement	1000	140	10	100	-	-	GI loss
Expected losses	1000	140	5	100			Third space
Nutrition					?	?	

2. Total requirements

3. Calculate replacement fluids

	H₂O	Sodium (Na)	Potassium (K)	Chloride (Cl)	Calories	Protein	Other
Oral, enteral nutrition							
Parenteral nutrition	1000	35	18	53	1000	4.25	(Standard TPN)
Specific replacement	1000	130	4	109	200	0	D5LR
Balance D5 1/2 NS	1000	77	0	77	200	0	

4. Total infusion

Simple starter:
D5 1/2 NS + 20KCl @ 1 cc/Kg/hr = 24 cc/Kg H_2O/day
 1.8 mEq Na/Kg/d
 0.5 mEq K/Kg/d
 4.8 cal/Kg/d

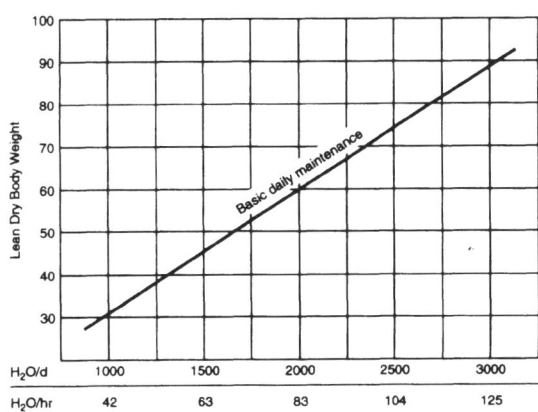

Nervous System

Level of Consciousness	Brain level	Glasgow Scale			Defect	
		Motor	Verbal	Eye	Metabolic	Anatomic
Alert, responds, opens eyes	All normal	6	5	4	—	—
Confused, disoriented	Cortex	5	4		—	—
Inappropriate words	Cortex		3		—	—
Eyes open to sound	Cortex			3	—	—
Withdraws to pain	Cortex	4			—	—
Makes sounds, no words	Cortex		2		—	—
Eyes open to pain	Cortex			2	—	—
Eyes closed, no response to sound	Midbrain		1	1	—	—
Decorticate (flexor) posture	Midbrain	3			—	—
Pupillary reflex	Midbrain				Present	Absent
Decerebrate (extensor) posture	Pons	2			—	—
Doll's eyes reflex	Pons				Present	Absent
Cold nystagmus reflex	Pons				Present	Absent
Flaccid to pain	Medulla	1			—	—
Spontaneous respiration only	Medulla				—	—

Cord levels	Sensory	Nerves	Motor
C4	Shoulder	—	—
C5	Outer arm	Musculocutaneous	Biceps
C6	Thumb	Radial	Extensors
C7	Middle finger	Median	Flexors
C8	Little finger	Ulnar	Interossei
T1	Inner arm	—	—
T4	Nipple	—	—
T10	Umbilicus	—	—
T11	Gonads	—	—
L1	Hip	—	—
L2	Thigh	Obturator	Adductors
L3	Knee	Femoral	Quadriceps
L4	Inner calf	Tibial	Gastrocnemius
L5	Big toe	Peroneal	Toe extensors
S1	Little toe	—	—
S4	Anal	—	Anal sphincter

Typical glasgow score range

Alert, awake, oriented, eyes open	15
Confused, speaks, opens eyes to sound	12
Unconscious but responds to stimulus (moves, opens eyes, makes sound)	10
Unconscious, withdraws or grimaces in response to pain	6
Unconscious, flexes in response to pain only	5
Flaccid	3

Head injury algorithm

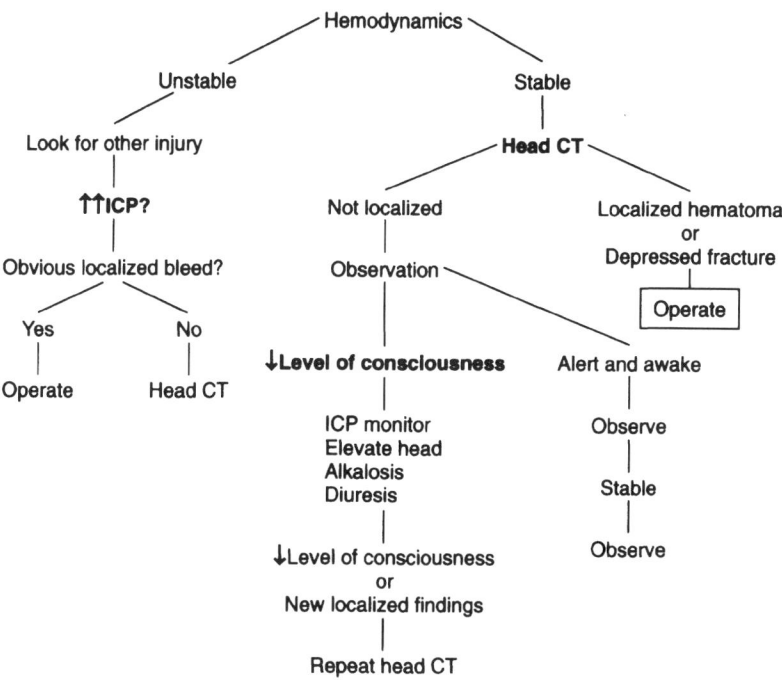

Seizure algorithm

Metabolic causes: hypoglycemia, hypoxia
Diazepam (Valium), 10–40 mg intravenously
Phenobarbital, 1 mg/kg intravenously up to 10 mg/kg total
Phenytoin (Dilantin), 500 mg intravenously up to 15 mg/kg total

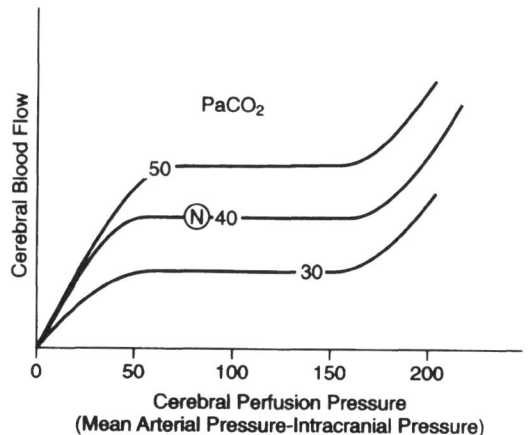

Host Defenses/ Coagulation

Coagulation/Thrombosis

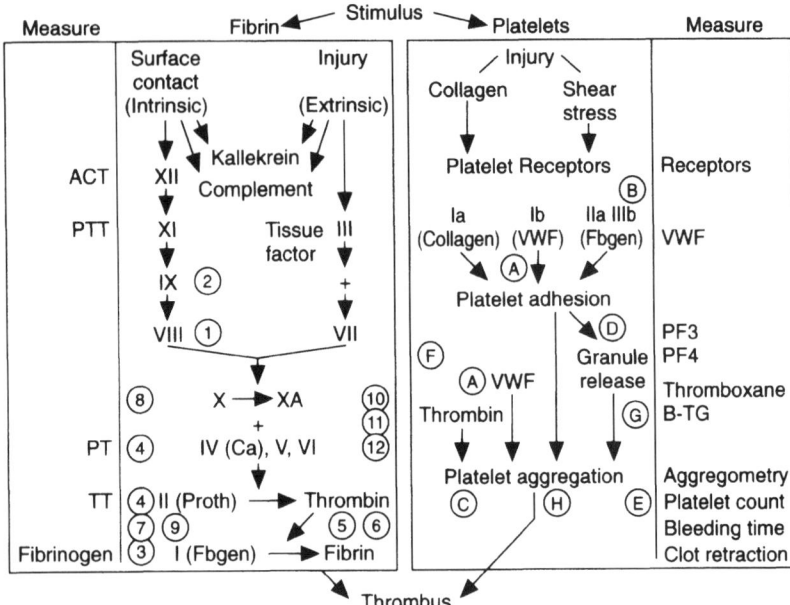

Diseases and drugs which slow/prevent:

Fibrin formation		Platelet function	
Factor deficiencies		Factor deficiencies	
VIII Hemophilia A	①	VWF	Ⓐ
IX Hemophilia B	②		
I Hypofibrinogenemia	③	Diseases	
		Glanzman's disease	Ⓑ
Diseases		(missing receptors)	
Liver failure II, V, VII	④	Renal failure	Ⓒ
Circulating FDP	⑤	(mechanism?)	
Hypothermia (slows all steps)	⑥	Surface exposure	Ⓓ
		CPB, ECMO, dialysis	
Drugs		(granule release)	
Coumadin	⑦	Thrombocytopenia	Ⓔ
Heparin (several steps)	⑧	Hypothermia (slows all steps)	Ⓕ
Hirudin	⑨		
		Drugs	
Normal inhibitors		Aspirin	
Thrombomodulin	⑩	Ibuprofen	Ⓖ
Protein C	⑪	Dipyridamole	
Protein S	⑫	PGI$_2$	Ⓗ

Typical patterns of coagulopathy*

	Platelet count	Bleeding time	Fibrinogen	PTT or ACT	PT	TT	FDP
External bleeding and transfusion	↓	↑	↓	↑	↑	↑	0
Internal bleeding and transfusion (very common)	↓	↑	↓	↑	↑	↑	↑
DIC (very rare)	↓	↑	↓	↑	↑	↑	↑
Thrombocytopenia	↓	N	N	N	N	N	0
Thrombocytopathia	N	↑	N	N	N	N	0
Liver failure	N	↑	↓	↑	↑	0	0
Hemophilia	N	N	N	↑	N	N	0
Coumadin	N	N	N	N ↑	↑	N	0
Heparin	N	N	N	↑	↑	↑	0
von Willebrand's disease	N	↑	N	N	N	N	0
Fibrinolysis	N	N	N	↑	↑	↑	↑
PRBC and saline	0	—	↓	↑	↑	↑	0
Frozen plasma	0	—	N	N	N	N	0
Platelets	↑	—	N	N	N	N	0

*Abnormal coagulation test results associated with various clinical conditions. Notice that the pattern for internal bleeding associated with transfusion and DIC is the same.

Bleeding management algorithm

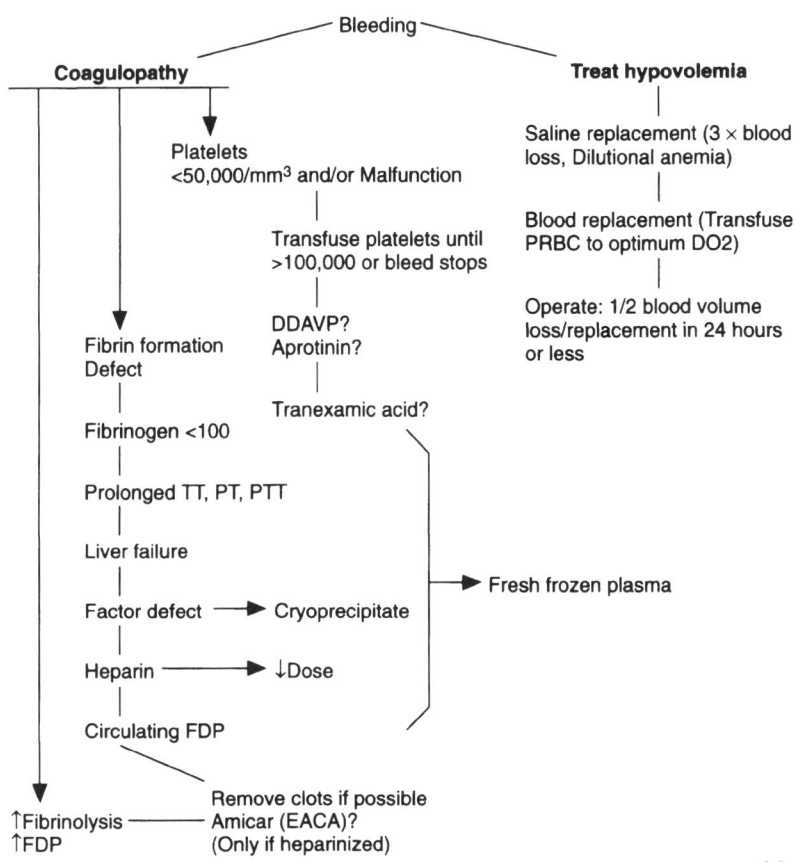

Host Defenses/Infection

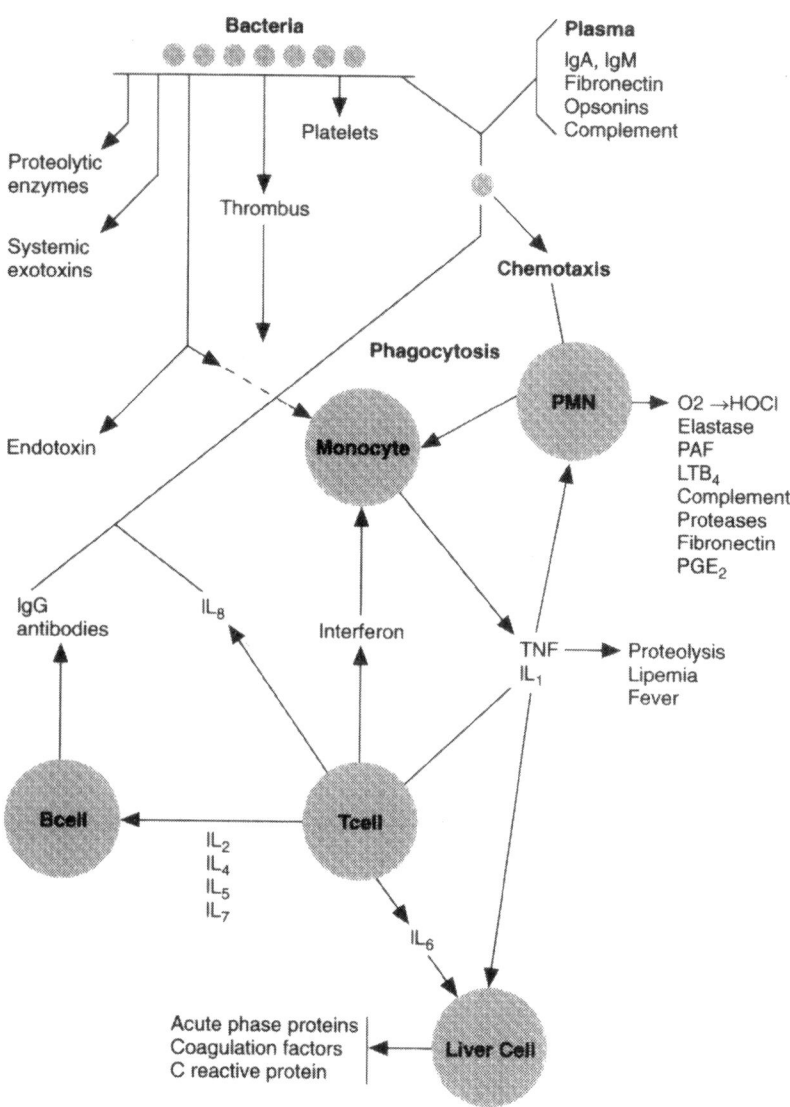

ICU antibiotic choices

Family	Antibiotic	IV Dose	Relative Cost/d	Staphcoag-	Staphcoag+	MRS	Strep A,B	Enterococcus	H flu	Bacteroides	Clostridium p	Common Gm-	Enterobacter	Pseudomonas	Serratia	Citrobacter	Acinetobacter
Penicillins	Pen G	2 mill q 4	10	●			●	o			●						
	Methicillin	1 gm q 4	30	o	●												
	Oxacillin	1 gm q 4	60	o	o												
Other Gm+	Vancomycin	.5 gm q 6	32	o	o	●	o	o									
Aminopens	Ampicillin	.5 gm q 6	16	o			o	●	●			o					
	Aztreonam	1 gm q 8	30									o		o	o		
Combinations	(Timentin)	3 gm q 4	54	o	o					o	o	o	o	o			o
	(Unasyn)	1 gm q 6	20	o	o					o	●	o					
	(Primaxin)	.5 gm qp 4	90	o	o					o	o	o	o	o	o	o	o
Macrolide	Erythromycin	.25 gm q 4	30	o	o		o										
Cephalosporin	Cephalothin (Keflin)	1 gm q 4	18														
I	Cefazolin (Kefzol)	1 gm q 6	24	o	o							o	o	●			
	Cefotetan (Cefotan)	1 gm q 12	20														
II	Cefuroxime (Zinacef)	1 gm q 8	24	o	o							o	o	o		o	
	Cefotaxime (Claforan)	1 gm q 8	30														
III	Ceftriaxone (Rocephin)	1 gm q 12	60	o	o				o			o	o		●	●	
	Ceftazidine (Fortaz)	1 gm q 8	42														
Anti Ps III	Cefoperazone (Cefobid)	1 gm q 8	30	o	o							o	o	●	●	●	
Aminoglycosides	Gentamycin	.08 gm q 8	6	o	o	o		o				●	●	●	o	o	●
	Tobramycin	.08 gm q 8	21	o	o	o		o				o	o	o	o	o	o
	Amikacin	.5 gm q 8	120	o	o	o		o				o	o	o	o	o	o
Other Gm-	Metronidazole (Flagyl)	.5 gm q 6	48							●	o						
	Trimethoprim sulfa (Bactrim)	.25 gm q 6	88	o	o							o	o			o	
	Clindamycin	.6 gm q 8	33							o	o						
	Chloramphenicol	1 gm q 6	16	o	o		o	o	o	o	o	o					
Quinoline	Floxin	.4 gm q 8	9	o	o	o			o			●	●	o	o	o	o
Antifungal	Amphotericin B	.05 gm q 24	27														
	Fluconazole	.2 gm q 12	20														
Antiviral	Acyclovir	1 gm q 8	240														
	Gancyclovir	.5 gm q 12	240														

o = Usually sensitive
● = Drug(s) of choice

Scoring Systems

Acute injury score (AIS-85)

	Head/Neck	Face	Thorax	Abdomen	Extremity	External
Score: Range:	0–5	0–5	0–5	0–5	0–5	0–5

Range: 0 = Normal, 1 = Minimal, 2 = Moderate, 3 = Severe but not life threatening, 4 = Severe and life threatening, 5 = Critical, survival is uncertain
LD50: Convert to injury severity score (ISS)

(From: The Abbreviated Injury Scale (AIS)—1985 revision. Des Plaines, IL: American Association of Automotive Medicine; I Civil, W. Schwab. The abbreviated injury scale, 1985 revision. A condensed chart for clinical use. J Trauma 1988;28:87–90.)

Injury severity score (ISS, Baker)

Score: square AIS for each region, then sum.
Range: 0 (normal) to 75 (arbitrary maximum).
LD50: 35.

	AIS	AIS^2
Example: Mild closed head injury	3	9
Ruptured spleen	4	16
Fractured femur	3	9
Total:		34 ISS

(From SP Baker, et al. The injury severity score: a method for describing patients with multiple injury and evaluating emergency care. J Trauma 1974;14:187–96.)

Trauma Score (Champion)

	Respiratory Rate	+ Effort	BP	Capillary Refill	Glasgow
Score:	0–4 0 = Critical High = Normal	0–1	0–4	0–2	1–5
Range:	16 (normal) to 1				
LD50:	10				

(From: HR Champion, W Sacco, TK Hunt. Trauma severity scoring to predict mortality. World J Surg 1983;7:4–11.)

Acute physiology score (APS, Knaus)

	Temp.	BD	HR	ABG	Na	K	Creatinine	Hct	WBC	Glasgow
Score:	0–4 0 = Normal 4 = Critical	0–4	0–4	0–4	0–4	0–4	0–4	0–4	0–4	0–12
Range:	0 (normal) to 48									
LD50: Convert to APACHE II										

Acute physiology and chronic health evaluation II (APACHE II, Knaus)

Score: APS + Age factor + Past history factor
Range: 0 (normal) to 56
LD50: 20 – 25

Glasgow coma score

Best motor response	Best verbal response	Best eye response	Score
Obeys			6
Localizes	Oriented		5
Withdraws	Confused	Spontaneous	4
Abnormal respiration	Inappropriate	To sound	3
Extensor respiration	Sounds	To pain	2
None	None	None	1

Range: 15 (normal) to 3
LD50: 8

The APACHE II severity of disease classification system (Knaus, 1995)

Physiologic Variable	High Abnormal Range				Normal	Low Abnormal Range		
	+4	+3	+2	+1	0	+1	+2	+3
Temperature, rectal (°C)	≥41°	39°-40.9°	—	38.5°-38.9°	36°-38.4°	34°-35.9°	32°-33.9°	30°-31.9°
Mean arterial pressure (mm Hg)	≥160	130-159	110-129	—	70-109	—	50-69	—
Heart rate (ventricular response) (beats/min)	≥180	140-179	110-139	—	70-109	—	55-69	40-54
Respiratory rate (nonventilated or ventilated) (breaths/min)	≥50	35-49	—	25-34	12-24	10-11	6-9	—
Oxygenation: AaDO$_2$ or PaO$_2$ (mm Hg)								
a. FiO$_2$ ≥ 0.5; record AaDO$_2$	≥500	350-499	200-349	—	<200	—	—	—
b. FiO$_2$ < 0.5; record only PaO$_2$	—	—	—	—	PO$_2$ > 70	PO$_2$ 61-70	—	PO$_2$ 55-60
Arterial pH	≥7.7	7.6-7.69	—	7.5-7.59	7.33-7.49	—	7.25-7.32	7.15-7.24
Serum sodium (mmol/L)	≥180	160-179	155-159	150-154	130-149	—	120-129	111-119
Serum potassium (mmol/L)	≥7	6-6.9	—	5.5-5.9	3.5-5.4	3-3.4	2.5-2.9	—
Serum creatinine (mg/dL) (Double-point score for acute renal failure)	≥3.5	2-3.4	1.5-1.9	—	0.6-1.4	—	<0.6	—
Hematocrit (%)	≥60	—	50-59.9	46-49.9	30-45.9	—	20-29.9	—
White blood cell count (Total/mm³) (in 1,000s)	≥40	—	20-39.9	15-19.9	3-14.9	—	1-2.9	—
GCS score = 15—actual GCS score.								
A Total APS. Sum of the 12 individual variable points.								
Serum HCO$_3$- (Venous—mmol/L) (Not preferred; use if no ABGs)	≥52	41-51.9	—	32-40.9	22-31.9	—	18-21.9	15-17.9

B Age points
Assign points to age as follows:
Age (yrs)	Points
≤44	0
45-54	2
55-64	3
66-74	5
≥75	6

APACHE II SCORE

Sum of **A** + **B**

A APS points _____

B Age points _____

C Chronic health points _____

Total APACHE II _____

AaDO$_2$ = alveolar-arterial gradient for oxygen; ABGs = arterial blood gases; APS = acute physiology score; FiO$_2$ = fraction of inspired oxygen; GCS = Glasgow coma score; PaO$_2$ = arterial oxygen pressure; PO$_2$ = partial pressure of oxygen.
From: WA Knaus, et al. APACHE II: A severity of disease classification system. Crit Care Med 1985; 13: 818-29.

C Chronic health points:
If the patient has a history of severe organ system insufficiency or is immunocompromised, assign points as follows:
a. For nonoperative or emergency postoperative patients—5 points, or
b. For elective postoperative patients—2 points.

Definitions:
Organ insufficiency or immunocompromised state must have been evident **prior** to this hospital admission and conform to the following criteria:
Liver: Biopsy-proven cirrhosis and documented portal hypertension; episodes of past upper GI tract bleeding attributed to portal hypertension; or prior episodes of hepatic failure/encephalopathy/coma.
Cardiovascular: New York Heart Association functional class IV.
Respiratory: Chronic restrictive, obstructive, or vascular disease resulting in severe exercise restriction, e.g., unable to climb stairs or perform household duties; or documented chronic hypoxia, hypercapnia, secondary polycythemia, severe pulmonary hypertension (>40 mm Hg), or respirator dependency.
Renal: Receiving chronic dialysis. *Immunocompromised:* the patient has received therapy that suppresses resistance to infection, e.g., immunosuppression treatment, chemotherapy/radiation, long-term or recent high-dose steroid therapy; or has a disease that is sufficiently advanced to suppress resistance to infection, e.g., leukemia, lymphoma, AIDS.

Multiple Organ Failure Adult ICU Patients

One organ failure only

	Mortality (%)
Respiratory	22
Renal	38
Liver	27
Cardiac	67
Infection	28

Concomitant organ failure

No. of organs	Mortality (%)
1 (Respiratory only)	40
2	55
3	75
4	80
5	100

(From: RH Bartlett. Critical Care Handbook, Ann Arbor: Department of Surgery, University of Michigan, 1993; RH Bartlett, et al. A prospective of acute hypoxic respiratory failure. Chest 1986;89:684–689.)

Systemic Inflammatory Response Syndrome (SIRS)

Concensus Conference Definitions

SIRS:
Temperature $>38°C$ or $<36°C$
WBC $>12/mm^3$ or $<4,000/mm^3$
Pulse >90 beats/min
Respiration >20 breaths/min
Sepsis
   SIRS negative culture
   severe, no shock
   severe, with shock
   SIRS positive culture
     severe, no shock
     severe, with shock

Mortality

Overall: 9% (1206 pts)
2 criteria 6%
3 criteria 9%
4 criteria 18%

10
16
46
16
20
46

(From: ACCP-SCCM: Definitions for sepsis and organ failure and guidelines for the use of innovative therapies in sepsis. Crit Care Med 1992;26:864; M Rangel-Fransto et al. The natural history of the systemic inflammatory response syndrome [SIRS]: a prospective study. JAMA 1995;273:117–123.)

ARDS Scoring Systems

ARDS/ALI definitions (Bernard, Concensus Conference, 1994)

1) Acute onset, 2) Bilateral infiltrates, 3) PCW < 18
plus $PaO_2/FiO_2 < 300 =$ Acute lung injury
    $PaO_2/FiO_2 < 200 =$ ARDS

Murray lung score (Murray, 1988)

X-ray study	PaO_2/FiO_2	Compliance	PEEP (cm H_2O)	Score	Approximate Mortality (%)
Normal	>300	>1.0	<5	0	0
1 quadrant	255–299	0.4–0.9	6–8	1	25
2 quadrants	175–224	0.4–0.7	9–11	2	50
3 quadrants	100–174	0.2–0.4	12–14	3	75
4 quadrants	<100	<0.2	>15	4	90

(From: JF Murray, et al. An expanded definition of the adult respiratory distress syndrome. Am Rev Respir Dis 1988;138:720–3.)

Geneva score (Morel, 1985)

X-ray Study	$AaDO_2/FiO_2$	Compliance	EIP (cm H_2O)	Score	Approximate Mortality (%)
Normal	<300	>1.0	<20	0	0
Interstitial	300–375	0.6–0.9	20–25	1	25
Interstitial	375–450	0.5–0.7	25–30	2	50
Consolidation	450–525	0.3–0.5	30–35	3	75
Consolidation	>525	<0.3	>35	4	90

(From: D. Morel, et al. Pulmonary extraction of serotonin and propranolol in patients with ARDS. Am Rev Respir Dis 1985;132:475–84.)

Euroxy study (Artigas, 1991)

X-ray Study	PaO_2 (mm Hg)	FiO_2	PEEP (cm H_2O)	Tidal Volume (cc/kg)	Score	Approximate Mortality (%)
Infiltrate	>75	0.5	5	10	Hypoxic	38
Infiltrate	<75	0.5	5	10	Severe	69

(From: A Artigas, et al. Clinical presentation prognostic factors and outcome of ARDS in the European collaborative study [1985–1987]. In: W Zapol, F Lemare, eds. Adult respiratory distress syndrome. New York: Dekker, 1991:37–63.)

Massachusetts General Hospital score (Zapol, 1991)

X-ray Study	Ventilation	Oxygen	Severity	Mortality (%)
Minimal	+/− Intubate	$FiO_2 < 0.5$	Mild	18
Panlobular	PPV	$FiO_2 > 0.5$	Moderate	49
Bilateral	PPV + PEEP	$FiO_2 > 0.6$ or $PaO_2 < 50$ mm Hg	Severe	84

(From: WM Zapol, et al. The adult respiratory distress syndrome at Massachusetts General Hospital. In: W Zapol, F Lemare, eds. Adult Respiratory Distress Syndrome. New York: Dekker, 1991:367–80.)

ICU class (UMMC SICU)

I: Unstable, ventilator, inotropic drugs, existing organ failure
II: Stable, ECG or pressure monitoring, high risk for organ failure
III: Stable, no special monitoring

Liver Failure (Child, 1960)

Class	Bilirubin (mg/dL)	Albumin (g/dL)	Ascites	Encephalopathy	Malnutrition
A	<2	>3.5	0	0	0
B	2–3	3–3.5	Mild	Mild	Mild
C	>3	<3	Severe	Severe	Severe

(From: CG Child. Hepatic circulation and portal hypertension. Philadelphia: Saunders, 1954.)

Pancreatitis (Ranson, 1974)

Admission findings	48 hour findings
Age >55 yr	Hematocrit ↓ 10%
Glucose >200 mg/dL	BUN ↑ 5 mg/dL
LDH >300 Iu/L	Calcium <8 mg/dL
SGOT >250 IU	PaO_2 <60 mm Hg
WBC >16,000/mm^3	BBD >4 mEq/L
	Fluid >6 L

(From: JAC Ransom, et al. Prognostic signs and role of operative management in acute pancreatitis. Surg Gynecol Obstet 1974;139–69.)

Positive signs	Mortality (%)
3–4	15
5–6	50
7+	80+

Myocardial infarction (Killip, 1967)

NYHA class	Cardiac failure	Ejection fraction	Mortality (%)
I	None	0.47	8
II	Mild	0.36	30
III	Pulmonary edema	0.31	44
IV	Cardiogenic shock	0.12	80+

(From: T Killip, JT Kimball. Treatment of myocardial infarction in a coronary care unit. A two-year experience with 250 patients. Am J Cardiol 1967;20:457.)

Critical Care Drug Doses

	IV Dose	Preparation	
Inotropes and Vasopressors			
Dopamine (Inotropin)	3–20 µg/kg/min	250 mg in 250 ml	15 gtts = 250 µg
Dobutamine (Dobutrex)	3–20 µg/kg/min	250 mg in 250 ml	15 gtts = 250 µg
Isoproterenol (Isuprel)	.01–1 µg/kg/min	2 mg in 250 ml	15 gtts = 2 µg
Epinephrine	.01–.01 µg/kg/min	2 mg in 250 ml	15 gtts = 2 µg
Norepinephrine (Levophed)	.01–.1 µg/kg/min	2 mg in 250 ml	15 gtts = 2 µg
Amrinone (Inocor)	5–10 µg/kg/min	5 mg in 250 ml	15 gtts = 5 µg
Phenylephrine (Neo-Synephrine)	2–5 µg/kg/min	10 mg in 250 ml	15 gtts = 10 µg
Ephedrine	25 mg IM or IV		
Methoxamine (Vasoxyl)	5 mg IM or IV		
Digoxin	.125–.25 mg/d	Load 1 mg, follow level	
Vasopressin (Pitressin)	0.1 IU/min IV	20IU/100 ml	
Anti-hypertensives and Vasodilators			
Alpha-blockers			
Phentolamine (Regitine)	.03–.3 µg/kg/min	50 mg in 250 ml	15 gtts = 50 mg
Hydralazine (Apresoline)	5–20 mg q 6 h	20 mg/ml	
Chlorpromazine (Thorazine)	1–5 mg q 6 h	50/2 ml	
Diazoxide (Proglycem)	50–300 mg	300 mg/20 ml	
Nitrates			
Nitroglycerin	.5–8 µg/kg/min	50 mg in 250 ml	15 gtts = 50 µg
Nitroprusside (Nipride)	.5–8 µg/kg/min	50 mg in 250 ml	15 gtts = 50 µg
ACE Inhibitors			
Captopril (Capoten)	100 mg q 6 h PO		
Enalapril (Vasotec)	5 mg q d oral		
Methyldopa (Aldomet)	100–250 mg q 6 h	50 mg/ml	
Beta-blockers (see Class II Antiarrhythmia)			
Calcium channel blockers (see Class IV Antiarrhythmia)			
Antiarrhythmia			
I (Fast Ca channel blockers)			
IA			
Quinidine	300–600 mg IV		
Procainamide (Pronestyl)	2–6 mg/min	2 gm in 250 ml	15 gtts = 2 mg
IB			
Lidocaine	200 mg IV, 1–4 mg/min	2 g in 250 ml	15 gtts = 2 mg
Phenytoin (Dilantin)	300–500 mg q 4 h		
II (Beta blockers)			
Propanolol (Inderal)	1–5 mg	3 mg in 10 ml	
Atenolol (Tenormin)	5–10 mg	5 mg in 10 ml	
Esmolol (Brevi bloc)	.5 mg/kg, .05 mg/kg/min	2.5 gm in 10 ml	
Metoprolol (Lopressor)	5–15 mg	5 mg	
III (Delay repolarization)			
Bretylium	500 mg × 3	2 gm in 250 ml	15 gtts = 2 mg
Amiodarone (Corodarone)	25–200 mg/d	oral	
IV (Slow Ca channel blocker)			
Verapamil (Isoptin)	1–5 mg IV	1 mg/ml	
Nifedipine (Procardia)	10 mg tid	oral	
Diltiazem (Cardizem)	.25 mg/kg/, 10 mg/h	25 mg/ml	
V (Other)			
Adenosine	6 mg IV × 5		
Digoxin	.25–.5 load, then 0.1 mg/d		
Bradycardia			
Atropine	.4 mg × 2		

Bronchodilators
   Xanthine
      Aminophylline   5 mg/kg, follow effect   500 mg/250 ml   15 gtts = .5 mg
   B-2 Agonists
      Terbutaline (Brethine)   .25 mg SQ, repeat   2 mg/2 ml
      Albuterol (Proventil)   2 puffs, 200 µg nebulized   Inhaler, 200 µg caps
   Inhaled steroids
      Beclomethasone (Vanceril)   2 puffs   Inhaler
Mucolytic
   Acetyl cysteine (Mucomyst)   1–3 ml q 4 h nebulized   20% solution
Diuretics
   Furosemide (Lasix)   20–200 mg IV q 6 h
   Ethacrynic acid (Edecrin)   20–100 mg IV q 6 h
   Bumetanide (Bumex)   .5–1 mg IV q 6 h
   Mannitol   25 gm IV q 6 h
   Acetazolamide (Diamox)   250 mg q 6–12 h   500 mg/10 ml
   Spironolactone (Aldactone)   50 mg qid PO   25 mg pills
Buffers
   Tris, Tromethamine (THAM)   50–250 mEq   18 gm (150 mEq)/500 ml
   Bicarbonate   50–250 mEq   50 mEq/50 ml vials
   HCl   50–250 mEq   .1 Normal (100 mEq/L)
Neuromuscular Blockers
   Depolarizing agents
      Succinyl choline (Anectine)   1–1.5 mg/kg
   Non-depolarizing agents
      Pancuronium (Pavulon)   .1 mg/kg   .3–.5 mg/kg/min
      Atracurium (Tracrium)   .3–.5 mg/kg   7–10 mg/kg/min
      Vecuronium (Norcuron)   .06–1.0 mg/kg   1 mg/kg/min
   Non-depolarizing reversal
      Neostigmine   2 mg × 2 IV   1 mg/ml
      Edrophonium (Tensilon)   10 mg IV   10 mg/ml
Analgesics
   Opiates
      Morphine   10 mg q 3–4 h   10 mg q 3–4
      Meperidine (Demerol)   100 mg q 3–4 h   100 mg q 3
      Fentanyl   100 mg q 1 h   100 mg q h
      Hydromorph (Dilandid)   1.5 mg q 3–4 h   1.5 mg q 3 h
   Antagonist
      Naloxone (Narcan)   1 mg, titrate   .4 mg/ml
Sedatives/Anesthetics
   Barbiturates
      Thiopental (Pentothal)   100–200 mg IV
      Phenobarbital   200–500 mg, follow effect T level   15–40 mg/ml
   Anesthetics
      Propofol (Dipravan)   2 mg/kg, 100 mg/kg/min   1000 mg in 100 ml
      Ketamine   3 mg/kg IV
   Benzodiazepines
      Diazepam (Valium)   5 mg IV   10 mg/2 ml
      Midazolam (Versed)   1–5 mg IV
      Lorazepam (Ativan)   1–5 mg IV
   Benzodiazepine Inhibitor
      Flumazenil (Romazicon)   .2 mg IV × 5   .1 mg/ml vial
   Neuroleptic
      Haloperadol (Haldol)   1–5 mg IV or IM   5 mg/ml
   Other
      Dilantin   300–600 mg follow effect T level   10–20 mg/ml
      Ethanol   100 ml/hr IV   5% Ethanol
GI Drugs
   H2 Blockers
      Cimetidine (Tagament)   300 mg IV q 6 h   300 mg/2 ml
      Famotidine (Pepcid)   200 mg IV q 12 h

Ranitidine (Zantac)	150 mg PO bid	
H+ Inhibitor		
Omeprazol (Prilosec)	20 mg PO qd	20 mg caps
Gastric motility		
Metoclopramide (Reglan)	10 mg IV q 8 h	10 mg/2 ml
Anti secretory		
Somatostatin (Sandostatin)	50 μg q 8 h IV, IV, 1M	200 μg/ml
Coagulation		
Heparin	300 units/kg IV for total anticoagulation	1000 units or 10,000 units/cc
Coumadin	10 mg loading dose, then titrate by PT	
Thrombolytic		
Urokinase	300,000 u/60 min	
Streptokinase	1.5 mill u/60 min	250,000 u/100 ml
T-PA	10 mg/2 min 50 mg/1 hr	
Antiprotease, Antifibrinolytic		
Aprotinin (Trasylol)	10^6 units IV, then 10^5 units/hr	
EACA (Amicar)	5 gm IV, then 1 gm/hr	5 gm/100 ml
Tranexamic acid (Cyklokapron)	10 mg/kg IV q 6 h	100 mg/ml
Platelet agents		
DDAVP (Desmopressin)	.3 μg/kg	4 μg/ml
Platelet Inhibitors		
Aspirin	600 mg PO qid	600 mg tabs
Dipyridamole (Persantin)	100 mg PO qid	50 mg tabs
Ibuprofen (Motrin)	400 mg PO qid	400 mg tabs
Sulfinpyrazone (Anturane)	200 mg PO bid	200 mg caps
Vitamin K (Aquamephyton)	2.5–10 IM/SQ	10 mg/ml
Hormones		
Adrenal steroids		
Hydrocortisone	25–50 mg IV/IM	50 mg/ml
Methyprednisolone (SoluMedrol)	20–200 mg IV	500 mg vials
Fludrocortisone (Florinef)	0.1 mg PO qd	.1 mg tabs
ACTH	25 units (V)/1M	
Levothyroxine (Synthroid)	50–100 μg/d	200/10 ml vials
DDAVP for D.I.	2–4 μg/d IV	4 μg/10 ml

Blood Products
  Whole Blood
    Not routinely available
  PRBC
    365 ml
    Hematocrit 65%
    O negative and type specific available for emergencies
  Platelets
    Random donor
      Dose: 50 ml
      1 unit will ↑ platelet count 5,000–10,000 mm^3
      Usually ABO and Rh compatible
    Single donor
      Dose: 200–300 ml
      6 × number of platelets as random donor
      24 hrs required
  Plasma
    FFP
      Dose: 250 ml
      No platelets
      Does have V, VIII
Plasma Proteins
Cryoprecipitate (AHG)
  10 ml has 1000 units
Factor VIII for mild hemophilia or von Willebrand's disease
Pooled factor VIII for severe hemophilia
5% Albumin; 5 g/dL
25% Albumin; 12.5g/50 ml

Phone Numbers

Intensive Care Units

_____ _____ _____
_____ _____ _____
_____ _____ _____

Patient Floors/Nursing Stations

_____ _____ _____
_____ _____ _____
_____ _____ _____

X-Ray

Portable _____   Angio _____   Schedule _____

CT Head _____   GI _____   Reports _____

CT Body _____   Bone _____

MRI _____   Chest _____   _____

_____

Labs

Chem _____   _____   _____

Hematol _____   _____   _____

Micro _____   _____   _____

Blood Bank _____   _____   _____

OR Desk _____   Schedule _____   Supervisor _____

Anesthesia _____   _____   _____

ER _____   _____   _____

Paging _____   Admitting _____   Security _____

Pharmacy _____   Nutrition Team _____

Resp. Therapy _____   Dialysis _____

On-call Rooms _____   _____   _____   _____

Made in the USA
Lexington, KY
08 March 2012